7 Day
BOOTCAMP
for Brides

7 Day Bootcamp for Brides
Tone It, Burn It, Bring It — Feel Fit, Focused And Fabulous On Your Wedding Day!

Anita Revel

© 2010

ISBN 978-0-9804439-7-4

AUSTRALIA

Published by Now Age Publishing Pty Ltd
PO Box 555, Cowaramup,
Western Australia 6284
NowAgePublishing.com

Cover by   Inspired Insight
inspired-insight.com

Cover image © LaraK via Fotolia

7 Day BOOTCAMP for Brides

ANITA REVEL

now age
PUBLISHING

Table of Contents

Bootcamp Basics

You're about to spend thousands of dollars on a dress, ceremony, reception and (gulp!) the wedding photographer. As the bride, you'll be the centre of attention, after all. So this is the one day of your life you want to be looking your best. Are you ready to be centre stage for your big day, looking and feeling beautiful for your friends, family and the wedding photos?

You're investing so much in every other aspect of your day, now it's time to invest the same energy in yourself. Do justice to the time and money you're pouring into your wedding day by turning up feeling fit, focused and fabulous. This guide will show you how to achieve this in just seven days.

Are you ready to look hot? Are you ready to look stunning in your gown as the epitome of the "glowing bride"? Are you ready to smile your way through your day with every detail taken care of, stress free?

Together with Coach Bridie (the bride on the cover of this book), we will guide and support you to become the glowing bride you want to be. Coach Bridie, you and I are about to spend seven whole days together seeking total reevaluation and rejuvenation. Be ready to give up any mental blocks, tired old excuses or physical hang-ups that get in the way between you and success, and promise you will give it every bit of attention that it (and you!) deserves.

Something old – You, as a stress-head

Something new – You, after this program

Something borrowed – My advice

Something WOO! –
Your guests' reaction when they see you!

Why 7 Days?

As a Civil Marriage Celebrant, I meet dozens of brides every month at various stages during their wedding planning. When I first meet with newly engaged couples, I often see the brides looking fresh, happy and on a high from their recent engagement. It's a different story when I meet them again for their wedding rehearsal a week out from their big day.

In my experience, brides are so busy organising a thousand details… from the time they are engaged, to the minute they arrive at the church, they are micro-managing their dream day. In all the chaos they forget about themselves. All too often the bride finds herself one-week out from her wedding with blotchy skin from stress and black bags under her eyes from lack of sleep.

The bride sometimes panics at this point. Bad habits emerge as she finds herself eating carrot sticks and drinking nothing but coffee and champagne. Stress levels rise, tempers shorten and high hopes plummet.

This is where my 7 Day Bootcamp for Brides helps. Sure it's not ideal to overhaul one's life in seven days, but considering the circumstances, this program is the most realistic and positive regime you can action right now.

The ideas and exercises outlined in this program have been developed by professional nutritionists and fitness coaches and motivational experts, so you can be assured the program being presented to you is the most practical and safe option for you right now. Furthermore, as it's so full of common sense you can apply the tools to daily routine for the rest of your life.

So give this program your best shot. You'll naturally regain your poise and glow as you follow the step-by-step tips throughout. Just think of it as seven days of eating, moving, breathing, and finding your sexy-sleek- chic-inner-goddess.

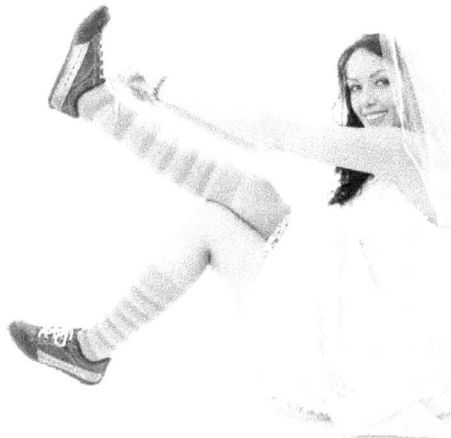

Bridie says...

The more I move, the more energy I have

What to Expect

Women have a spirit, energy, and attitude that deserves to be nurtured. We generally have natural gifts of emotional intelligence and intuitive wisdom… this powerful drive within us can be used to propel our physical well-being. It's a Catch 22 situation, though. Both systems – body and attitude – need to be mutually nurtured for lifelong holistic well-being. That is why this bootcamp focuses not only on "diet and exercise" but also on harnessing the power of your mind.

According to a survey of 1,000 brides by Fitness magazine, 83% wanted to shed weight before their wedding, and many were prepared to take drastic action to achieve their goal.

It's pointless working out, sweating and starving your body if you haven't aligned your attitude to one of self-appreciation and success. With the wrong attitude the workout simply becomes a routine of self-punishment.

To make the exercise and nutrition components of this program infinitely easy to do, you will be required to adopt a healthy attitude. I will show you how to do this, not only throughout the duration of this bootcamp, but as you enter upon a very important new stage in your life; your marriage.

Creating a Healthy Body

Your body is your vehicle for living the rest of your life. Your body belongs to only you, and is your one unique feature that separates you from over six billion other people. Your body is what your soon-to-be-spouse will desire every day, and yes, your body is only as old as the attitude you have towards it.

The 7 Day Bootcamp For Brides focuses on healthy eating and exercise, and how the combination of real food, recreation and rest benefits your body. You will be able to take these tips with you as a resource for lifelong health.

Getting Your Attitude in Gear

You probably know from experience how powerful your mind is and how it can affect your physical body. When we stress or become mentally fatigued, for example, our immune system reacts by weakening and making us more vulnerable to illnesses. Furthermore, we develop a lack of self-confidence which in turn results in low salary expectations, under-developed relationship skills (both personal and professional), and a feeling of "missing out" in all the good stuff other people seem to enjoy.

When you can see and tweak your attitude to a healthy one – one that lets you see the good in you and your world – then you can really enjoy the nutrition and exercise offered in this program. You will find a new joy in treating your body like the sacred vessel it is. You are going to bring it the day of your wedding with a,"Hey yeah, I'm here to rock it."

Keeping Track of Accomplishments

When sticking to an exercise and nutrition program there is nothing more motivating than seeing your achievements in black and white. Journaling is great for this – it helps you keep track of your achievements *and* it keeps you honest. For example, it's pretty sobering to have to admit, "Dear diary… today I baked my girlfriend a chocolate mud cake. Then I had to bake another one because I ate the first one while watching an entire season of *Sex and the City* for 12 hours straight."

In other words, if you commit to journaling your every move and morsel, you'll be more inclined to stick with the program. Your journal doesn't need to be a guilt trip confession box, but a confidant where you can write down food and drink intake, what type of exercise you did and for how long. Include any thoughts, hopes, feelings and experiences. This is a place for testimony, laughter, and pride in yourself. You'll look back on it after your wedding and be thankful you gave this gift of time and energy to yourself.

There is space in this book for you to journal as you go, but you can also use a notebook, wedding journal, an online fitness journal, your blog, or even an iPhone application – there are plenty to choose from.

Call on the Cheer Squad

Your cheerleaders are those people who surround you, and who love and support you. Having strong pillars of support will determine how well you adapt to healthy changes, maintain your self-confidence, and keep on a path of success.

Your mind and willpower need to be fuelled by outside encouragement to become even stronger and more confident.

It would be awesome if you could find an accountability partner (or two or three) during this time that will keep you going and focused. They will keep the voices of opposition away from you while encouraging others to cheer you on as well. Any kind of change in your life may cause you to feel vulnerable, and as you prepare for your wedding, you need supports from all sides.

Gather your cheer squad up and share your intentions about this program and your goals. You can even suggest making these healthy changes common goals for all of you, so you can keep each other motivated along the way. Your cheerleaders have nothing but unconditional love for you, and will lift you with praise as you approach your wedding day with a stronger body and mind.

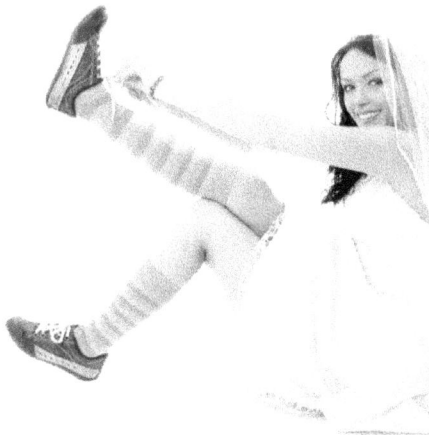

Bridie says…

Just for this week, stay away from any friends who encourage you to smoke, drink, over-eat and sloth

Excuses, Excuses

Fair enough, you're busy and have responsibilities. For some of us cramming every moment with an activity is what we thrive on. It helps keep our minds off the really important stuff, like… pampering ourselves, giving time to our true passions, resolving past hurts, revelling in our brilliance… Ah, but it all comes down to choice. Here are some ways you can choose to combat the most common excuses…

I have no time

This boot camp program is so full of common sense advice you won't even know you're doing it. It is no-fuss enough to incorporate into your week so you can focus on what may feel like innumerable other responsibilities.

If you feel like fitting the fitness portion of this program will be a struggle to squeeze with your other pre-wedding responsibilities, at least make the most with what you have. Fitness doesn't have to be a segmented part of your day. You can always do squats while brushing your teeth, lunges while walking from one place to another and bicep curls while you're on the phone. Just keep it top of mind to keep moving.

My friends make me drink champagne

As Coach Bridie says, just for this week, stay away from any friends who encourage you to smoke, drink, over-eat and sloth. If this is impossible, at least hydrate before you de-hydrate (and during!) by drinking lots of water. (See the chapter on re-hydration.)

I'm too stressed

Here are five ways to beat the wedding stress blues.

1. **Touch Therapy**. Get touched in some way, such as a hug, a foot or back massage – anything that activates your body's relaxation response in charge of reducing your stress-causing hormones.

2. **Meditation**. Focus on your breathing patterns to allow oxygen to flow to your vital organs. This will help you relieve tension, sharpen your awareness and concentration, and reduce stress. Yoga is an awesome outlet for this. Affirmations and mirror work are also great, which we'll explore later.

3. **Delegate Tasks**. Forget being in control of every little detail. Determine honestly what could be done, at least in part, by someone else. Give away some of the wedding tasks so you can focus on your health.

4. **Eat Right**. Food has a direct link to stress. The right food can lower stress, the wrong food makes you cranky and flighty. Reduce caffeinated and alcoholic beverages, and eliminate fried and processed food.

5. **Focus on your relationship**. Nothing can put strain on a relationship more than excess stress, and your focus right now is your relationship with your fiancée. Exercise together, go to a spa together, spend time together. When you make time for exercise, involve him. He probably could use exercise as a stress reliever as much as you!

In Summary

The 7-Day Bootcamp for Brides focuses on the two main areas that encompass your health holistically: your body and your attitude.

Each day, Coach Bridie and I encourage you to spend equal time honouring that beautiful body of yours, and learning to change your attitude to one of self-appreciation – really learn to love your awesomeness.

The Bootcamp will give you the foundations of great nutrition, enjoyable exercise and attitude adjustments that you will be able to apply to your routine for the rest of your life.

Give this program everything you've got. If you say, "I'll try it out, maybe it will work," you'll get corresponding results. Instead, give 100 percent to your success and unleashing your inner wow-factor.

Step By Step – Your Bootcamp Companion

Let's avoid aimless meanderings and detours and cut to the chase – to be successful with the *7 Day Bootcamp For Brides*, it helps to have a checklist to guide you.

> If you don't know where you want to finish up, then any road will get you there.
>
> ~ Lewis Carroll (via the Cheshire Cat).

Seven days' worth of checklists are provided over the page. Tick each box as you complete each task. Fill in details of activities – how much you did of what, and for how long. Make notes about where you can improve, what your triggers were for success or failure, and how each activity made you feel. Carry this book with you everywhere you go so you can write down your food and fitness achievements the second you do them.

How to Use Your Companion

The Tasks	My Journal	Time
Real Food eaten today	Record every morsel of food that passes by your lips. Writing it down makes you more accountable for the food choices you make. If you're absolutely honest with yourself, knowing you'll be writing down the "12 chocolate chip cookies" will, ideally, make you think twice about eating them. This is also a great way to ensure you're eating at the right times and in the right combination for the most efficient supply of energy for your metabolism.	Meal times, calories, emotion, energy highs and lows
Recreation done today	This is a starting point for working out how many calories you've burned to compensate for any extra treats consumed during the day. It is also a way to make sure you find the time to schedule in exercise, whether it be a structured workout (intentional) or taking the stairs instead of the lift (incidental).	Did you cover the "treats" with extra exercise?

cont...

The Tasks	My Journal	Time
Rest time taken today	Again, this is designed to make sure you schedule time for *you*. Make yourself and your rejuvenation a priority. Describe the kind of rest you had, or the type of pamper time you took.	Success?
Attitude adjustment	Start every day with a healthy stretch. Make it the first thing you do when you get out of bed. Stretch your body, your arms, your legs, even your fingers and jaw. During this time you can think about which affirmation you'll be using today, which theme song is going to rock your socks. You might also think about which tasks you can delegate to make your week easier. Follow this with a "Mirror Work" activity of your choice. No matter what, make "I am kind to myself" your number one rule.	Will you take this skill with you for the rest of your life?

Day One

The Tasks	My Journal	Time
Real Food eaten today	☐ Breakfast: ☐ Morning tea: ☐ Lunch: ☐ Afternoon tea: ☐ Dinner: ☐ Other:	
Recreation done today	☐ Yoga: ☐ Intentional exercise: ☐ Incidental exercise:	

cont...

Rest time taken today	☐ Awake time: ☐ Rest taken during the day: ☐ Bed time: ☐ "Me Time" taken today:	
Attitude adjustment	☐ Morning stretch ☐ Mirror work ☐ Affirmation: ☐ Today's theme song: ☐ Things delegated today	

Day Two

The Tasks	My Journal	Time
Real Food eaten today	☐ Breakfast: ☐ Morning tea: ☐ Lunch: ☐ Afternoon tea: ☐ Dinner: ☐ Other:	
Recreation done today	☐ Yoga: ☐ Intentional exercise: ☐ Incidental exercise:	

cont...

Rest time taken today	☐ Awake time:	
	☐ Rest taken during the day:	
	☐ Bed time:	
	☐ "Me Time" taken today:	
Attitude adjustment	☐ Morning stretch	
	☐ Mirror work	
	☐ Affirmation:	
	☐ Today's theme song:	
	☐ Things delegated today	

Day Three

The Tasks	My Journal	Time
Real Food eaten today	☐ Breakfast: ☐ Morning tea: ☐ Lunch: ☐ Afternoon tea: ☐ Dinner: ☐ Other:	
Recreation done today	☐ Yoga: ☐ Intentional exercise: ☐ Incidental exercise:	

cont...

Rest time taken today	☐ Awake time: ☐ Rest taken during the day: ☐ Bed time: ☐ "Me Time" taken today:	
Attitude adjustment	☐ Morning stretch ☐ Mirror work ☐ Affirmation: ☐ Today's theme song: ☐ Things delegated today	

Day Four

The Tasks	My Journal	Time
Real Food eaten today	☐ Breakfast: ☐ Morning tea: ☐ Lunch: ☐ Afternoon tea: ☐ Dinner: ☐ Other:	
Recreation done today	☐ Yoga: ☐ Intentional exercise: ☐ Incidental exercise:	

cont…

Rest time taken today	☐ Awake time: ☐ Rest taken during the day: ☐ Bed time: ☐ "Me Time" taken today:	
Attitude adjustment	☐ Morning stretch ☐ Mirror work ☐ Affirmation: ☐ Today's theme song: ☐ Things delegated today	

Day Five

The Tasks	My Journal	Time
Real Food eaten today	☐ Breakfast: ☐ Morning tea: ☐ Lunch: ☐ Afternoon tea: ☐ Dinner: ☐ Other:	
Recreation done today	☐ Yoga: ☐ Intentional exercise: ☐ Incidental exercise:	

cont…

Rest time taken today	☐ Awake time: ☐ Rest taken during the day: ☐ Bed time: ☐ "Me Time" taken today:	
Attitude adjustment	☐ Morning stretch ☐ Mirror work ☐ Affirmation: ☐ Today's theme song: ☐ Things delegated today	

Day Six

The Tasks	My Journal	Time
Real Food eaten today	☐ Breakfast: ☐ Morning tea: ☐ Lunch: ☐ Afternoon tea: ☐ Dinner: ☐ Other:	
Recreation done today	☐ Yoga: ☐ Intentional exercise: ☐ Incidental exercise:	

cont…

Rest time taken today	☐ Awake time: ☐ Rest taken during the day: ☐ Bed time: ☐ "Me Time" taken today:	
Attitude adjustment	☐ Morning stretch ☐ Mirror work ☐ Affirmation: ☐ Today's theme song: ☐ Things delegated today	

Day Seven

The Tasks	My Journal	Time
Real Food eaten today	☐ Breakfast: ☐ Morning tea: ☐ Lunch: ☐ Afternoon tea: ☐ Dinner: ☐ Other:	
Recreation done today	☐ Yoga: ☐ Intentional exercise: ☐ Incidental exercise:	

cont…

Rest time taken today	☐ Awake time:	
	☐ Rest taken during the day:	
	☐ Bed time:	
	☐ "Me Time" taken today:	
Attitude adjustment	☐ Morning stretch	
	☐ Mirror work	
	☐ Affirmation:	
	☐ Today's theme song:	
	☐ Things delegated today	

Notes

_____

_____

_____

_____

_____

_____

_____

_____

_____

_____

_____

_____

_____

_____

_____

_____

_____

_____

_____

_____

_____

_____

Fundamentals for Awesomeness: The Four Rs

Each day you will be required to keep track of four essential aspects of a healthy body, also known as the Four Rs:

1. Real Food,
2. Recreation,
3. Re-Hydration (more on this later) and
4. Rest.

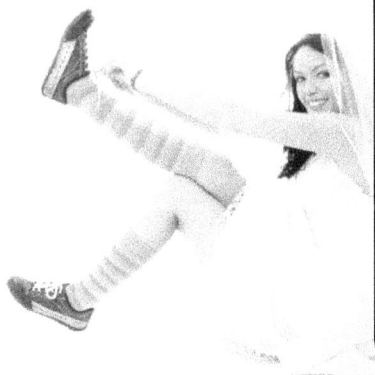

The "Body" part of the bootcamp is based on these Four Rs. Journal these each day to ensure you keep it all in balance – great food, plenty of H20, enjoyable exercise and heavenly repose.

1. Real Food

Choosing real food is as simple as dividing food into two food groups – processed and unprocessed, or natural and unnatural. Eating real food, rather than processed food or fast food, is your priority during this bootcamp.

Of course you will be tempted to eat on the fly as you run from appointment to appointment; you will be offered endless canapés and finger foods as you swan from one pre-wedding party to the next; and you will probably find yourself reaching for the nearest snack food to throw down your throat in between phone calls.

Resist, resist, resist. Have fresh fruit in a bowl on the table. Cook up a large batch of vegetable soup and freeze individual portions for emergencies. Make rounds of sandwiches and freeze them – you'll be able to reach for them at a moment's notice when hunger pains hit.

If your goal in this program is to lose a dress size (and to find your "thinner goddess"), you will need to abide by the rules of science and intake fewer calories than you can burn off. Note, fewer calories does not mean foregoing yummy food. It just means wiser choices in your food selection. If you do slip and indulge in "Un-Real Food" there are two things you must do:

✓ Forgive yourself and move on;

✓ Increase your "Recreation" time. We will get in touch with the calorie tango in a moment, along with the most important rule: eat the goodness you want to feel.

2. Recreation

There are two types of people in this world: those who are born to exercise, and those that can't be bothered. For the next seven days, put yourself in the former category. Be bothered and the results will be well worth the effort.

In Australia, national guidelines recommend 2.5 hours of moderate exercise a week – this works out to around 30 minutes a day. The United States Department of Agriculture goes one step further and recommends 60 minutes a day to prevent weight gain, and up to 90 minutes to help with weight loss. Here are some unique ways to exercise without the pain:

- ✓ Adding just 2000 more steps to your day can prevent weight gain, says Dr James Hill at the University of Colorado Health Sciences Center. Walk your dog to the furthest tree for his wee, walk on the spot while watching TV, or pace while talking on the phone.

- ✓ Burn more fat on your treadmill by exercising in walk-jog-walk cycles of one minute each. You'll get a longer, easier workout than had you run flat-out from the start to the finish.

- ✓ Encore! Pretend you're the conductor of an orchestra. Their 'wing-flapping' motions give them an awesome cardiovascular workout.

- ✓ Become Sir Dance-a-Lot. How is it that James Brown didn't die at 27 like Jimi Hendrix, or at 21 like Sid Vicious? With his never-ending high-kicks, air-jumps, mid-air splits and energetic whoops into the mic, James did the equivalent of a step class at every performance.

3. Re-Hydration

Yes, you've heard it all before – you must drink around two litres of fresh water a day. Don't under-estimate the value of this advice – water is necessary to nourish your skin, organs, mind and attitude. It fills out your wrinkles (or 'laugh lines' as modern goddesses call them) and makes your skin glow.

4. Rest

While your current life may be crazy and mad busy, I can't reiterate enough how important it is to grab 30 minutes of "Me Time" every day. Without it, you remain a slave to your routine, to others' demands and in the loop of stress. Stress causes our adrenal glands to release a hormone called cortisol.

Cortisol "…makes us store fat in case of famine," says David Cameron-Smith, Associate Professor in Nutrition Sciences at Deakin University in Melbourne.

So, stress = cortisol = fat storage. It also gives us a jelly belly as the fat gain tends to sit around the abdomen. The solution is to increase your exercise, recreation and Me Time to spark the release of beta-endorphins – brain chemicals which improve mood and promote calm. As such, Me Time prevents jelly belly.

Sleep is another important thing to do. Sleep deprivation can increase the hormone that stimulates appetite (ghrelin), and decrease the hormone that makes us feel full (leptin). So get lots of zeds to help produce more leptin – not only does it suppress your appetite, but the rest recharges your batteries and rouses you to get active.

Real Food Rules

The Real Food Rules are based on no starving, no sacrifice; just four great tools for eating well to stay well.

The following four rules will see you losing a dress size without any effort. All you need to do is stick with them!

1. Eat slowly,
2. Complement your foods,
3. Eat early, and
4. Detox and cleanse

It's only seven days – you can do it. Ideally they'll become habit-forming, in which case, welcome to life-long health.

> Three apples a day will give you 15 grams of fibre – this is half the daily recommended intake.
>
> They are also awesome for extending your metabolic rate. Add them to your shopping list.

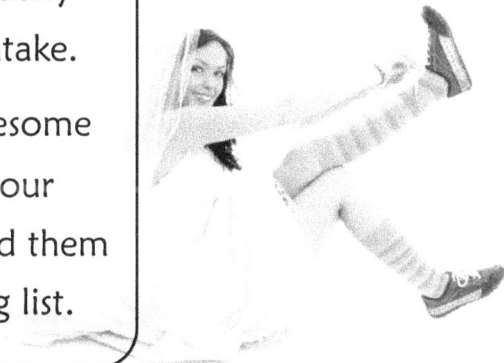

1. Eat Slowly

Avoid overeating by eating slooowly. Stretch receptors in your stomach tell your brain when you're hungry and you need food, and when you're full. This is great, but it takes twenty minutes for the message to get from your stomach to your brain before you register that you're full. By eating slowly, your body has more time to register the "You're full!" message and you'll ultimately eat less.

Also help your body by checking out actual recommended serving sizes – they are generally half of any restaurant meal. Set that portion aside, and pack, hide, store all of the rest of the food. You just want to sense that you are full. It's simple, and you won't need to measure your food, go hungry or feel deprived, and you will mentally feel satisfied.

> Try serving food on your smallest plates and in smaller bowls and glasses.

2. Complement Your Foods

The food plans included in this bootcamp have been created purposefully for their vitamins and nutrients, calorie counts, and fat/carb content. Furthermore, each meal is made up three essential elements:

1. Protein (meat, eggs, cheeses, some nuts)
2. Good Carbs (vegetables, pasta, bread and grains)
3. Good Fats (olive oil, avocados, sesame seeds etc)

Balancing these three elements will keep your body fuelled efficiently. You won't get energy highs or lows, your insulin will stay in check, and your metabolism will behave beautifully keeping you fuller for longer. The rule of thumb is 30/60/10:

- ✓ 30 percent of your meal should be protein,
- ✓ 60 percent carbohydrates (mostly vegetables) and
- ✓ 10 percent good fats.

More on Carbs

Breads, pastas, starches (like white potatoes) are all types of carbs, and they do serve beneficial purposes for our body by supplying glucose, proteins, and fats.

Although you don't need to jump on the no-carb diet fad, through personal experience I have learned that carbs are best when consumed during the earlier part of your day when you can burn off the sugar surge that carbs provide. If you waited until dinnertime, the sugar will less likely be burned, and turn into fat.

Also, wild or brown rice, whole grain breads and pastas are a great alternative to their white grain counterparts, because "white" grains, "white carbs" contain simple sugars that are easily broken down. Once food is broken down, you feel hungry again. Whole grain oatmeal, toast, whole grain pitas are all going to make you feel fuller longer, because brown carbs made of complex sugars take a longer time to be broken down. You will have more energy without having to eat.

Wheat contains a protein called gluten, a common food allergen. For many people it is difficult for the digestive system to break gluten down which results in fatigue, bloating, and inhibited absorption of other vital nutrients. Cut wheat out of your diet to help eliminate bloating and allow your food to be digested properly.

3. Eat Early

Give your body a chance to burn your evening meal effectively and eat dinner three hours before you go to bed. If you go to bed routinely at 10:30pm, you need to have finished eating by 7:30. This will give your body enough time to digest – otherwise, whatever has not been digested will go to fat.

A further advantage is that you will be hungry for the most important meal of the day – breakfast – the favourite meal of skinny chicks. (*Skinny Chicks Don't Eat Salads: Stop Starving, Start Eating... And Losing!* Christine Avanti, Rodale Books, 2010).

You'll further enhance your trim-down efforts by trimming down your meal sizes throughout the day: huge breakfast, medium-sized lunch and a small dinner. Keep your metabolism burning evenly throughout the day with snacks such as an apple, half-a-dozen almonds or carrot sticks. Crunchy snacks in particular are great for promoting the endorphins – the feel-good hormone.

4. Detox and Cleanse

If you're like me, you've got to have your daily fix of caffeine, chocolate and possibly a glass of wine or two. Sadly, these vices dehydrate your body, irritate your bladder, and aggravate your stress and nervous system. So, for the next week they are off the menu.

Ideally, allow three days to overcome any withdrawal symptoms while detoxing. If you still need a coffee fix, try ½ decaf, ½ caffeinated coffee one day, and then switch to pure decaf coffee the following day. Think of it as going "warm turkey" to overcome headaches and fatigue gently.

Here are some other ways to improve your healthy glow:

✓ Got a party season ahead? Avoid temptation by postponing detox plans until after any major parties.

✓ Stock up on fruit, vegetables and herbal teas such as peppermint, camomile, ginger or green tea.

✓ Get yourself a jazzy water bottle and keep it attached to your hip. Having water on hand (and hip) makes it easy to increase your daily water intake to the magical two litre ideal.

✓ Breakfast may be half a grapefruit, an orange and a slice of watermelon. Lunch can be a salad with baby spinach and vegetables high in water content (think cucumber and tomato). Dress salads with olive oil. Go the brown rice for larger meals and load up the steamed vegetables.

Some other painless ways to eliminate toxins include:

✓ Eat fibre. Fibre reduces your hunger, helps colon function and eliminates toxic and other wastes.

✓ Remove temptation. Keep any fatty foods out of sight. Store treats in ceramic jars, or better still, leave them out of your shopping trolley to start with.

> If you are pregnant, unwell, or have a heavy dependency on foods, drinks, tobacco, or illegal drugs, please consult your general practitioner for advice.

Real Food Recipes

The following recipes are suggestions… of course if you have your own favourite (healthy) recipes go ahead and substitute. Bear in mind **portion control**…

Professor Wahlqvist (*Food and Nutrition*, Allen and Unwin, 2002) recommends a daily intake of protein of 0.75g per kilogram (.026 oz per 2.2 pounds) for a sedentary individual. So if you're inactive and weigh 70kg (150 pounds), this means 52.5g (1.8 oz) of protein – in other words, your steak should be around the size of the palm of your hand. Even a tin of tuna provides 80 percent of your daily requirement.

Basic ingredients you can choose from for each meal:

	Protein	Carbs	Good Fat
Breakfast	Egg(s), Bacon, Yoghurt	Fruits, Wholegrain toast	Sunflower seeds, grapeseed oil
Lunch	Tuna, Smoked salmon, Cheese	Salad, Crispbread, Whole bread, Rice crackers	Pepitas, Almonds, Avocado, Olive oil
Tea	Meat, Poultry, Fish	Vegetables, Brown rice, Rice noodles	Omega-3 in fish

Snack
Attacks

Green tea for its anti-oxidants

Edam cheese on a rice cracker

Air-popped popcorn

Almonds

Apple

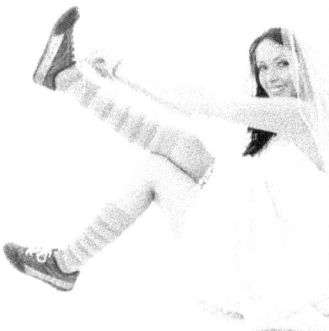

> In order to abide by the "Rest" rule, avoid the following food types that are know to sabotage sleep: chocolate, preserved and smoked meats, energy drinks, spicy foods and chili, and alcohol.

Examples of Great Recipes

The following combinations are examples of beautifully balanced meals. Stick with these and you will not feel hungry for the five hours in between each meal, nor will you experience the three o'clock slump during this time. These recipes can also be made gluten-free, by the way – a double win.

Shopping List

_____

_____

_____

_____

_____

_____

_____

_____

_____

_____

_____

_____

_____

_____

_____

_____

Breakfast

Vegetable Omelette

Whisk two eggs with some water, seasonings of your choice and a handful of finely chopped up vegetables – broccoli, mushrooms, baby spinach and capsicum is a tasty combo. Pour a drizzle of grapeseed or olive oil into a frying pan, then your egg mix. Cook on low heat until the top of the omelette begins to set. Fold in half and serve. An alternative is the Spinach and Bacon Omelette. Add crumbled turkey breast, 1 cup baby spinach, ½ cup chopped tomato and Feta.

Fruit Yoghurt Smoothy

Blend together five tablespoons yoghurt, one diced green apple, a handful of flaxseed, five almonds, and your choice of another piece of fruit: kiwi, fresh strawberries or frozen berries. You might choose to avoid bananas because of their high Glycemic Index, but use your intuition and ask your body what it needs. Pour the mix into a bowl and sprinkle with sunflower seeds.

Breakfast Burrito

In a bowl combine 3 eggs, 1 capsicum (bell pepper), ¼ cup diced red onions, ½ cup shredded cheese, ¼ cup sliced mushrooms, and ½ chopped tomato. Heat and scramble the mix in a large non-stick skillet. Heat a multi-grain tortilla by letting it sit on top of the egg mix on the stove for a second. Add the mix into the tortilla, sprinkle with cheese, roll up and enjoy.

Lunch

Smoked Salmon (or Cheese) Crackers

Spread four gluten-free crispbreads with a quarter of a mashed avocado. Sprinkle with finely chopped sugar snap peas, red capsicum, almonds and sesame seeds.
Lay no more than 20g of smoked salmon or low-fat cheese over each crispbread and garnish with a generous helping of sprouts.

Greek Salmon Salad with Lemon

Grill 100g (4 oz) salmon until it is fully cooked. In a bowl, combine three cups of romaine or similar dark leaved greens, ½ cup each diced tomato and cucumber and a crumbling of feta cheese. Top with the salmon, squeeze lemon over the bowl, and top with a balsamic vinaigrette.

Quesadillas

Heat up your skillet or griddle, drizzle with olive oil and lay down one tortilla. Sprinkle the cheese, add the protein source of your choice (such as cooked minced chicken or de-veined and cooked shrimp/prawns), top with ½ cup each of black beans, mushrooms and bell pepper, and top it with another tortilla. Fold the tortilla in half, giving the heat just enough time to toast the half it's already laying on, and then take a spatula, and carefully flip it. You may need to help it stay folded. Once the cheese melts, it's ready to eat. Easiest to cut with a pizza cutter.

Apple Almond Crunch Salad with Shrimp

Throw together in a bowl 100g cooked prawns (4 oz of cooked shrimp), 3 cups of dark mixed salad greens, ¼ cup of diced red onion, 12 almonds, 1 chopped cucumber, 1 whole diced apple, ¼ cup of shredded Edam cheese and 2 tbs of Italian vinaigrette.

Chicken Kebabs

Stick a mix of the following ideas onto skewers and grill until the chicken is fully cooked: chopped boneless skinless chicken breast, red capsicum (bell pepper) cut into wide strips, thickly sliced zucchini, red onion sliced into wide strips.

Your Own Favourite

_____

_____

_____

_____

_____

_____

_____

_____

_____

_____

Dinner

Baked Ginger Fish and Vegetables

Whisk together grated fresh ginger, a crushed garlic clove, one tablespoon sweet chilli sauce and two tablespoons each of gluten-free soy sauce and mirin. Place a salmon steak in the centre of a piece of foil and spoon marinade over each steak. Top with thinly sliced shallots and a slice of lemon. Wrap the fish in the foil and place it on a baking tray in a pre-heated oven at 220°C and bake for 15 to 20 minutes.

While this is baking, steam some 1cm thick slices of butternut pumpkin for 10 minutes or so, and half a bunch of bok choy for five minutes. Alternatively, steam the vegetables of your choice, or chop up raw capsicum, carrots and sugar snap peas.

To serve, remove the fish from the foil and place in a shallow bowl. Pour juices from the foil parcels over the top, and serve with the pumpkin and bok choy.

Roasted Lemon and Rosemary Chicken

Heat oven to to 425 F / 218 C. Baste one chicken quarter with a drizzle of olive oil, and sprinkle with salt and pepper. Cover with tin foil, and bake until cooked.

Remove foil, sprinkle with lemon juice and fresh rosemary, and bake for another ten minutes to crisp the outside. Serve with a side salad or as many steamed veggies as you can handle.

Fried Rice and Chicken

Wash a cup of wholemeal rice and simmer it in two cups of boiling water until *al dente*. Leave the rice to cool while you cut up a chicken breast (skin off) and a variety of vegetables such as shallots, broccoli, snow peas, zucchini, capsicum, corn kernels and so forth.

Lightly coat the bottom of a wok with olive oil and seal the chicken. Once it is browned, add the vegetables and stir-fry for a few minutes. Add the rice to the wok and toss all the ingredients until they are warmed through. Add chilli and herbs to suit and drizzle a measure of gluten-free soy sauce and mirin until the rice is lightly coated. Remove from heat and stir through roasted almond slivers. Serve with a sprinkling of sesame seeds and garnish with sprouts.

Your Own Favourite

_____

_____

_____

_____

_____

_____

_____

_____

_____

_____

Other Recipe Ideas

_____

_____

_____

_____

_____

_____

_____

_____

_____

_____

_____

_____

_____

_____

_____

_____

_____

_____

_____

_____

_____

_____

Recreation

The workout herein was created by Melanie Grace, a Perth (Australia) based personal fitness trainer. Bridal trainers, (trainers who work with women specifically for their wedding day), focus on areas like arms and shoulders, waist, abdomen, legs, and butt, because these target toning areas feature in your wedding dress.

> The best remedy for a slow metabolism is a long walk – toning up is literally a "walk in the park"!

In a program as short as this seven day program, it is not possible to create the type of ripped abs and defined biceps that feature on late-night infomercials, but we can sure tone up and refine your line.

It can be tempting to overdo the exercise on the first day – the adrenalin is high and your intention is super-charged. Do moderate how much exercise do (especially if you haven't done it for ages) and keep it within a safe, comfortable zone for you. Initially, short regular stints several times a day are better than one longer flat-out session each day – your muscles will have a better chance to acclimatise to their new demands.

Seeing Exercise and Food in Motion

To work out how much exercise you need, relate it back to how much food you're eating… Imagine your food intake and your exercise tally has to balance on your body's profit-and-loss sheet at the end of the day.

Remembering that > is the symbol for "is greater than", here is the rule of thumb:

- ✓ Food In = Energy Out (ideal).

- ✓ Food In > Energy Out = Weight Gain.

- ✓ Energy Out > Food In = Trim Down, Tone Up.

For example, if it takes 116 minutes of walking to burn off a bucket of french fries, get your Food In = Energy Out balance by finding a fast food joint that's a two-hour return journey on foot. (Everything is in walking distance if you have the time.)

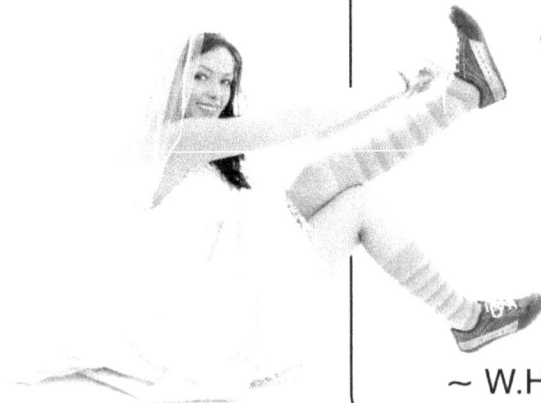

> Now shall I walk
> or shall I ride?
>
> "Ride,"
> Pleasure said.
>
> "Walk,"
> Joy replied.
>
> ~ W.H. Davies.

Guide: Walking for Weight Loss

Food	Quantity	Minutes walking*
Cup vegetables	1 cup	9 mins
Banana/apple	1 medium piece	25 mins
Pizza	1 slice	40 mins
Coke	375mL (large can)	41 mins
Potato Crisps	50g packet	68 mins
Mars bar	60g	72 mins
Sausages	150g	85 mins
Hot chips	225g (1 cup)	116 mins
Meat pie	1 individual	125 mins
Chocolate	100g	140+ mins
Chops	2	170+ mins

* 'Minutes of Walking' is based on a moderate pace that causes a slight, but not noticeable, increase in breathing.

If you can talk easily while walking, you could probably push up your walking speed a notch. If you can sing while you're walking, you're probably annoying your fellow walkers!

Guide: How to Burn Calories Quick

Activity	Calories/hour*
Sitting in the car	85
Budgeting (what?!)	90
Standing in queues	100
Driving	110
Dancing in your seat	180
Walking, 5kph	280
Tennis	350+
Skating/blading	420+
Shaking your booty	420+
Cycling, easy does it	450+
Jogging, 8kph	500
Swimming fast	500+
Running after kids	500+
Hiking	500+
Step Aerobics	550+
Rowing	550+
Power Walking	600+
Cycling fast	650
Squash	650+
Skipping with rope	700+

* Approximate

Target the Wedding Dress: the Workout

Equipment Needed to BRING IT

These are some tools that will benefit your workout experience a little more, without breaking the bank.

- ✓ Supportive shoes and proper apparel
- ✓ Yoga mat
- ✓ 2 kg - 4.5 kg hand weights
- ✓ Resistance band

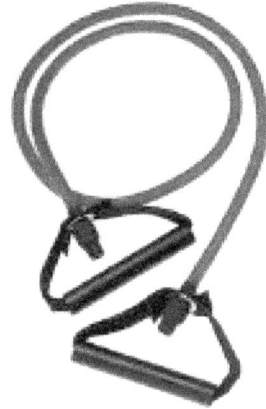

Find your Target Heart Rate

To work out your Maximum Heart Rate (MHR), deduct your age from 220. That is, if you are 24, your MHR would be 220–24 = 196.

Your Target Heart Rate should be between 65–80% of your MHR. For an MHR of 196, your target is between 127 –186 beats per minute.

Hint: Count your heart beats for 15 seconds and multiply the result by 4.

Warm-Up:

Squat Lift, Created for the total body workout.

Equipment Needed: Resistance band and dumbbells

1. Take your resistance band and secure it waist-high in the door – the door handle may be the right height for this.

2. Stand with your feet shoulder width apart, with your hands linked out in front your body to counterbalance your weight travelling backwards.

3. Sit down as though sitting on a small stool behind you, keeping your heels on the ground. Make sure your knees never come over your toes through the whole move. Bring your butt down to a point where your thighs are parallel with the ground.

4. Push up through your heels, making sure your belly-button is gently switched on (like you are drawing your belt one notch tighter).

5. Stand on your tip toes, and pull the cords even higher. Come back to the start.

6. Do this again for a total of 20 times.
    Inhale when you squat down,
    exhale when you come up.

This warm-up stretches your arms, shoulders, abdominal, and lower body muscles.

Arms

Hammer Curls with Weights

Stand with your feet apart, facing forward, and rest your arms by your sides holding the weights, palms facing in. Bring your forearms up to your chest, turning your palms inward to face your body. Pretend you are squeezing something in your elbow to contract those biceps Lower your arms. Remember to breathe in on the way down, and out on the way up.

20
repeats

Side Curls

Stand with your feet apart, facing forward, and rest your arms by your sides (with elbows slightly bent), holding the weights, palms facing your body. Lift the weights up to your shoulders, squeeze your muscles, and then lower the weights all the way back down.

15
repeats

Tricep Dips

Have a seat on a dining room chair or the couch and place both hands on either side of your hips with the fingers facing forward. Keep your feet flat on the floor in front of you. Bring your bottom off the chair, lover it toward the ground bending your elbows to a right angle at the back. Your elbows should be bending behind you, not to the side like wings.

15
repeats

Seated Dumbell Shoulder Press

While still seated, press your back to the chair. Sit up tall, feet flat on the floor, knees bent at a right angle, and bring dumbells to should level with your palms looking forward. From here push the dumbells up overhead but on a slight angle forward. Don't lock your elbows. Remember to breathe!

10 -15 repeats

Amazing Abs

Leg Extensions

Lay on your back, and with your arms straight by your side. Pull your knees towards your chest, your lower spine curling towards your head and tighten your abs. With one knee still by your chest, straighten the other leg as you lower it back towards the floor (without letting your heel touch the ground). Slowly control it as bring it back in towards you. Repeat with the other leg.

10 repeats

Leg Salutes

Lay on your back with your arms straight by your side. Lift both legs up towards the sky as if to salute the sky. Lower them down slowly, only letting your heels touch the ground on your last rep.

10 repeats

Side Planks

Lie on your side with your elbow directly underneath your shoulder. Stack your feet on top of each other and make sure your entire body is straight. Lift your torso off the ground so you are holding yourself up with your elbow and your knee (level 1) or your foot (level 2). If you choose level 1 bend your knees at a right angle. Contract the side of your trunk to hold you up and keep the bellybutton gently pulled towards your spine the entire time. Remember not to hold your breath.

30 - 60 seconds

Rotating Crunch-Peddle Pushing

Lay on your back with your knees bent at a right angle (feet off the floor). Cradle your head with your hands and keep the elbows in a straight line. Take one shoulder (whilst keeping the elbows in that straight line) towards the opposite knee whilst the other heel extends away from you to just above the ground. Keep alternating sides. Bring the head all the way back down to the ground in between each repetition. Slow and controlled is the key. Breathe out on the up and in on the way down

20 repeats

Hips

Standing Side Kick

Stand with your feet slightly apart with your hands on your hips. Lift one leg out to your side with your toe pointed outward, and then lower it back down. Do the same with the other leg. When you lift the started leg again, face your toe outwards (foot bent 90 degrees), and then lower it back down. Do the same with the other leg.

20 repeats

Side Jumps

Stand with your feet slightly apart, knees slightly bent, with your hands on your hips. Bend one knee up slightly towards your chest, and jump out about three feet to the side. Bring that foot down to the floor, and do the same with the other leg.

20 repeats

Hip Raise

Lay on your back with your knees bent, feet flat on the floor, and arms by your side. Lift your hips into the air, and extend your left leg, pointing your toe towards the wall. Hold this for one second, and then turn your leg (still straight) towards the side as close to a 90 degree angle from your body as you can. Hold for one second and return it to the front.

10 repeats

Squat Kicks

Stand up straight with your hands in fists up by your chest (think karate). Kick one leg up in the air, balance it up, and lower the standing leg into a squat. Return the other leg to the ground. This is a high powered activity.

15
repeats

Leg Raises

Spread out the yoga mat and get on all fours. Extend one leg out, the bottom-side of your foot facing the sky. Hold it for one second, lift six inches and hold for another second, and then return it to starting position.

Do the same with your other leg.

15
repeats

Butt

Heel Press

Lay on your back with your heels on a sturdy bench or the armrest of a couch. Keep your elbows bent at a 90 degree angle so that you are fully supporting your body. Lift your butt off the ground by pressing your feet into your support. Your upper body should be straight. Squeeze your glutes tightly, and lift one leg out to the side so it's perpendicular to your body, and then bring it back and lower yourself back down.

10
repeats

Chair Squats for Sexiness

Note: You don't have to start with weights – work your way up to them. With your weights held slightly above each shoulder, spread your legs shoulder-width apart, bend them slightly, and lower into a squat. Burn baby burn.

12
repeats

Walking Lunges

Start with your feet together and take a long step forward (still keeping the feet hip-width apart). Drop the back knee down towards the ground without letting the front knee come over the front toes. The back knee and the front knee should come down to a perfect right angle. The push back to the top should always come through the front heel (to get right into your butt!!) The next step forward comes from the opposite leg. Keep alternating legs.

20
repeats

Hip Extensions

Roll out the yoga mat, and get on your hands and knees. You actually want to be supported by your elbows and forearms. With the bottom of your foot facing the sky, kick your knee out, and hold it up in the air for two seconds. I know, I'm mean.

20
repeats

Re-Hydration

Drink lots of water to flush toxins from your vital organs, cary nutrients to your cells, moisten ear, nose, throat and eye tissues, and – here's the clincher – plump out your wrinkles to help you look younger.

It is generally accepted that eight glasses (two litres) of water a day is the ideal amount to keep you adequately hydrated, although a multitude of studies have proved varying suggestions over the years. No single formula fits everyone, so knowing more about your body's need for fluids will help you estimate how much water to drink each day.

I don't buy into the arguments – I just know what is right by my body by the condition of my skin (a longer term sign of success), how alert I'm feeling and, (an easy method), by the colour of my urine. It only takes a glance to gauge whether you're hydrated or dehydrated – your wee should be the colour of light straw. If it is dark yellow or gold, you are dehydrated.

> If the wee is clear, never fear
> If it's the colour of straw, drink some more
> But if it's the colour of gold, drink three-fold

It is really important for you to stay hydrated with the right fluids that will not only keep you energised, but feeling really good also. According to Jim Karas, New York Times Bestseller and author of *The 7 Day Energy Surge* (Rodale Books), here are the drinks you should have more of and the drinks you should avoid.

Drink More	Drink Less	Drink NONE!
Water	Coffee	Diet soda
Soup (homemade)	Milk	Regular soda
Tea (not high in	Protein shakes	Fruit juice drink
caffeine)	Canned soup	Energy drinks
Wheatgrass juice	Alcohol	Cordial
	100% pure fruit	
	juice	

The Easy Way to Get 8 Glasses a Day

This little excerpt comes from my illustrated eBook: *BOTIBOTO, Beautiful On The Inside, Beautiful On The Outside, A Self-Empowerment Story for Well-Rounded Women.*[1]

In the story, the heroine, Zenna, finds eight very easy ways to get eight glasses of water intake per day.

Try these ways to super-hydrate yourself effortlessly. Copy them into your journal and tick each idea off each time you have a glass. Alternatively, identify ways you will be able to fit in a glass here and there and add that to your list.

---

[1] *BOTIBOTO* is downloadable from Goddess.com.au

To drink eight glasses of water a day, get in the habit of drinking:

☐ A glass upon rising;

☐ A glass at breakfast;

☐ A glass before leaving the house for work;

☐ A glass upon arriving at work;

☐ A glass at morning tea;

☐ A glass at lunchtime;

☐ A small bottle of water to sip at the red traffic lights on the way home; and

☐ A glass while preparing dinner.

It's true. Zenna drinks around eight glasses of fresh water a day to nourish her skin, organs, mind and attitude. It fills out her wrinkles (or 'laugh lines' as modern goddesses call them) and makes her skin glow.

This is how easy it is to drink eight glasses of water a day for healthy skin:

- *A glass upon rising*
- *A glass at breakfast*
- *A glass before leaving the house for work*
- *A glass upon arriving at work*
- *A glass at morning tea*
- *A glass at lunchtime*
- *A small bottle of water to sip at the red traffic lights on the way home*
- *A glass before dinner*

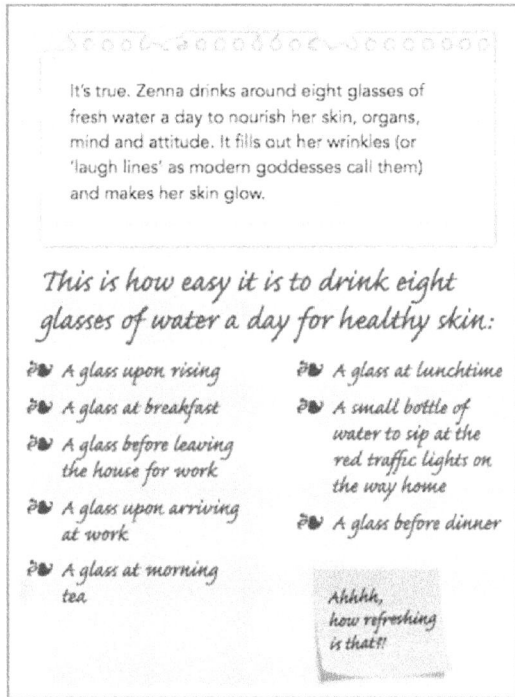

Ahhhh, how refreshing is that?!

Pssst. For an alternative to drinking water, try snacking on watermelon, tomatoes and cucumbers — these are between 90 – 95 percent water by weight.

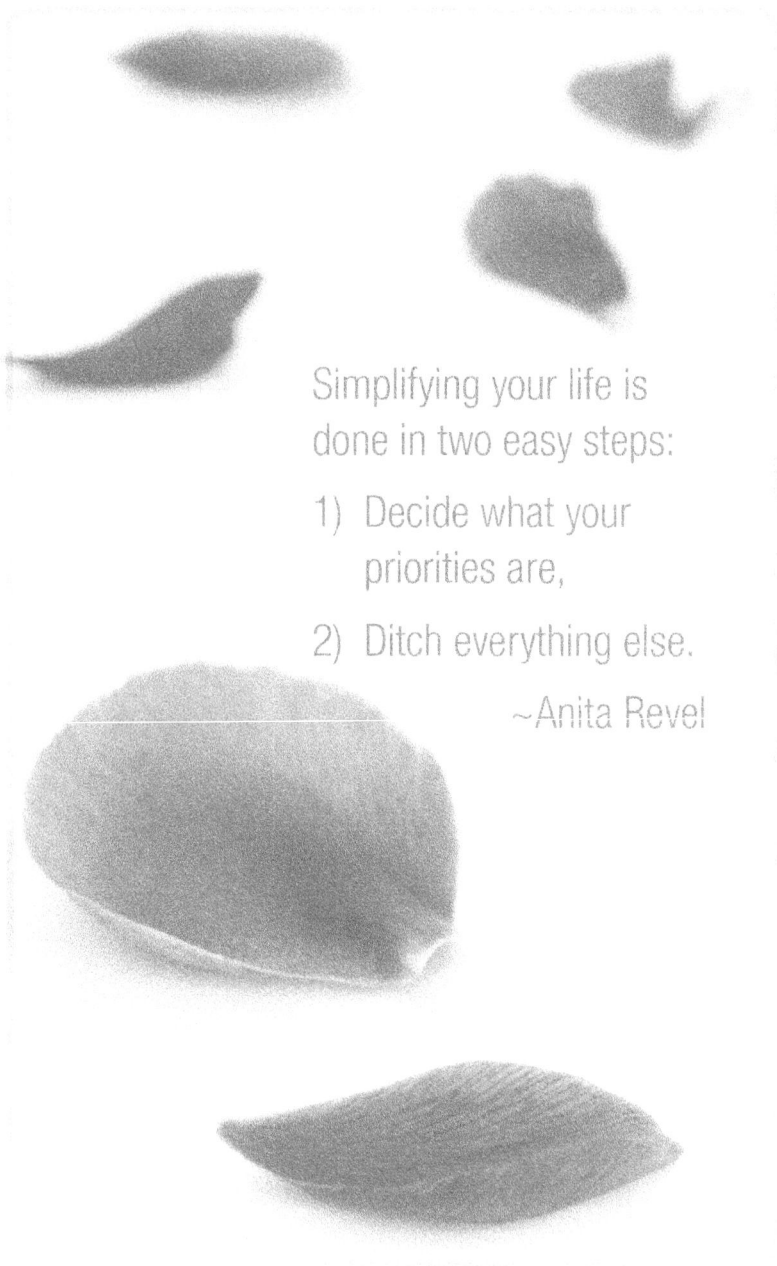

Simplifying your life is
done in two easy steps:

1) Decide what your
   priorities are,

2) Ditch everything else.

~Anita Revel

Rest

Taming the Inner Stress-head

Stress exacerbated by adrenaline, lack of sleep, PMS, caffeine overdose, all fuel your inner stress-head. You know she is stirring when your heart feels like it is burning or hurting, or there is churning in the pit of your stomach that makes you miserable. Sadly, she causes us to be brutal on ourselves and other people. The bad news is that the more you stress the more you feed and encourage her. But here is the **good news**… she is completely manageable with a few simple tools and techniques for quietening the mind and turning down the inner critic.

Stress = Weight Gain

The stress response, also known as the fight or flight response, is caused by an imbalance between your chaotic environment and how well you think you can handle it with what resources you have.

When you feel helpless, angry and directionless, these stress reactors cause your body to go into defence mode. Your adrenal glands kick in and release adrenaline and cortisol that give you bursts of energy to help you "flee" any perceived danger. When your body revs up those hormones it causes you to expend more energy than necessary for a very short time. As a result, your body reacts by immediately conserving energy and storing up fat by adding fats, sugar and insulin into your bloodstream. This cocktail makes it virtually impossible for you to lose weight.

Hence, the importance of being calm and happy in the lead up to your wedding. We'll be using two strategies to combat this: **Rest** and **Self-Appreciation**.

Calm the Savage Beast

As women we feed that little inner stress-head far too much… Even you, in the lead-up to what should be the happiest day of your life, are probably stressing about work, about where money is coming from, making your relationship with your fiancée work, getting your head around being married for life, eating right, sleeping right, finding negatives in yourself about yourself, raising children if you have children, worrying about yesterday, worrying about tomorrow, and good Lord, the wedding!!! Oh yes, wedding planning really gets the gold medal for being a stress initiator. Craaaaaaaaaaaap!

The inner stress-head is roaring… and taking it out on your body – here comes the three dastardly **bl**ahs: the **bl**ack bags, the **bl**oating and the **bl**otchiness. When you stress constantly, when you worry that nothing is going right, when you don't like yourself, you are causing your adrenals to go into overdrive, and then even in the calm, your brain can't make those hormones turn off. Stress also shuts down your digestion, reproduction, and even your immune system to save energy. This is why stomach ulcers, skipped menstrual cycles, and your vulnerability to viruses and germs is so prevalent in those who stress so much.

Literally, by letting your inner stress-head get the upper hand, you are sabotaging your success. The best way to tame this savage stress-head is to learn stress reduction techniques. Here we go…

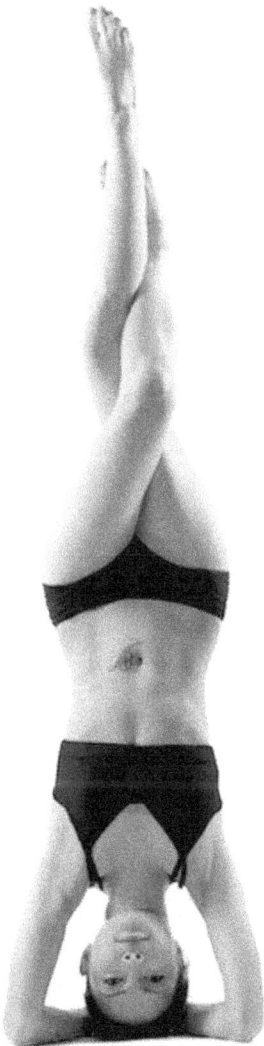

Breathing

Working with your breathing technique is one of the most effective, but yet most simple ways that you can embrace the calm. It is your body's natural relaxation response.

The simplest way to "breathe" is to close your eyes and consciously breathe in deeply through your nostrils, then releasing your breath in a controlled manner out your mouth.

Yoga workouts are particularly good for focusing on slow, rhythmic breathing – in fact, yoga is primarily a combination of stretches, balance, and breathing, and this combination initiates your relaxation response. Find a quiet, tranquil place, turn on some calming music, and consciously focus on slow, deep breathing for ten minutes.

Fidget!

Your brain, the electrical circuit of your body, may be running a hundred miles an hour. When you fidget, tap your feet, chew gum, run, jog, walk, swim – anything that requires constant movement, be it at your desk at work to a full-out exercise – you are giving your body a way to release pent up stress. Tap your feet more, tap your fingers on your body (your pressure points react and can help you relieve stress), wiggle your toes, do anything that will redirect your stress.

Find Your Quiet Voice

Our own inner voice is both a state-of-mind combined with feelings of the heart and positive mindset; it's the core (sane!) part of us which is responsible for our inner drive, our self-confidence, our logic, our love and ability to be intimate with another person… it is the voice that tells you, "You can do it!" and the sense of peace that washes over you when everything feels right in your world. It is normally not loud. It is graceful; it is beautiful; it is the still small voice inside of you that maintains tranquility, control, trust and inner strength.

I say it's quiet, because to be loud is to be speaking over something else – like what our heart or head does when we feel the need to cry and yell. To hear it and trust it, give up the noise from the rest of the world that belittles you or causes stress and anxiety. Focus on that voice inside of you that fosters total balance in your life. The more you can tune out the stressors in your life, the easier it will be to trust in yourself, and hear what your common sense says to do.

That still small voice can tame the inner stress-head. When your beast is roaring, look for your own body's guidance in the matter. Look within for answers. You already know what the right thing to do is in any given situation, it is simply a matter of trusting this inner voice – your intuition, if you will.

Trust Your Intuition

Some people call this inner quiet voice of reason, your intuition. Intuition is your body's natural wisdom that knows what is right or wrong for you. When you can learn to trust your intuition, you can stop fretting over making decisions – your inborn wisdom is telling you exactly the right way to go.

The first step in trusting your intuition is learning how to hear or feel your intuition. For some people it is a voice, for others a sense, and for others a physical reaction. Sometimes it's all three at once. If you are new to listening out for your intuition, here is one very simple way to hear or sense it…

The technique? Tossing a coin. Yep, tuning in to your intuition can be that easy. Here is how to do it:

1. Think of a question that can only have a **yes** or a **no** answer;

2. Hold the coin in your hand and assign **yes** to heads and **no** to tails;

3. Toss the coin and check the result – is it heads or tails? (And therefore, is the answer to your question, yes or no?)

When you see your answer represented by either heads or tails, feel what your body is doing. Is your gut churning? Is your heart jumping with excitement? Is a voice wailing "Noooo!" or is it singing "Yes!"? Or perhaps you are itching to toss it again until you get a different answer? If you're feeling disappointed then you know the true answer to your question – the opposite to how the coin landed. But if your head is singing "Yes!" then you also know the true answer to your question – it is according to how the coin did land.

The truth is, the coin didn't give you your answer. *You* did. You simply used the coin as a tool for understanding your intuition, and from your intuition you got your decision. If you're ever feeling overwhelmed this week, give yourself a break and resort to tossing a coin for your answer.

Time-Out and Yoga

Meditation and yoga are ways to connect with the divine and devote just a short period of time where your brain and body can take a break. They also decrease muscle tension, lower blood pressure and heart rate, increase alertness and let you connect with your inner wow-factor. Let your mind wander. acknowledge your blessings – all the things you have got to be grateful for. Give thanks for the support you've received to this day. Think about what a great catch you are!

Even if you can't set aside 30 minutes to meditate or do yoga each day, at the very least lay on a mat, arms out-stretched, and melt into the floor. Lower your respiration and heart rate, and just be in the moment. Simply… *be*.

Simple Yoga Guide

The suggested yoga poses are from my book, *The Goddess DIET, See a Goddess in the Mirror in 21 Days*[2], and were devised by Natalie Maisel, a yoga teacher, moon mistress and workshop leader based in California. Natalie is inspired by goddess energy in certain yoga positions and associated ritual and affirmations, which she shares via her website[3]. I love Natalie's work because she actively and reverently teaches that yoga is a wonderful practice for helping women to see themselves as the goddesses they are and were created to be.

On a physical level, yoga is wonderful for promoting health because "the asanas, or postures, are beneficial for every Goddess-y part of you to lengthen your muscles, increase bone density, cultivate flexibility, encourage toxin elimination, promote blood flow and circulation, open the joints, release stale, stuck energy and emotions, and to cleanse and detoxify your organs."

Daily life brings with it the normal everyday challenges and triumphs, but "… yoga helps to restore each women to her supreme glory and recognition of herself. Allow this ancient practice to transform your life on every level: physical, mental and emotional," recommends Natalie.

You will find seven simple poses described and illustrated over the page. If you're unfamiliar with yoga, *please seek professional assistance* to reap the benefits of proper practice.

---

[2] www.TheGoddessDiet.com

[3] www.GoddessDownload.com

Warrior II / Athena

As you hold your posture, increase the effectiveness with this chant, "Conceive it, believe it, take aim to achieve it, let go to Athena, prepare to receive it"!

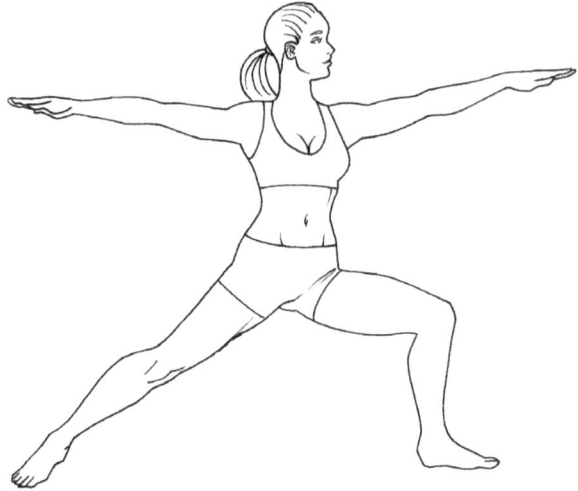

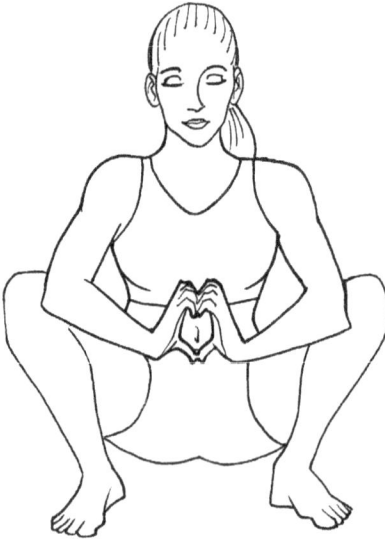

Garland Pose / Aphrodite

This is a variation of the Garland Pose, with the hands placed over your naval – the location of your sacral chakra.

As you hold your posture, call on Aphrodite with this chant, "Aphrodite, Aphrodite, come to me, fill me with passion and creativity".

Utkatasana / Chair / Fierce Pose

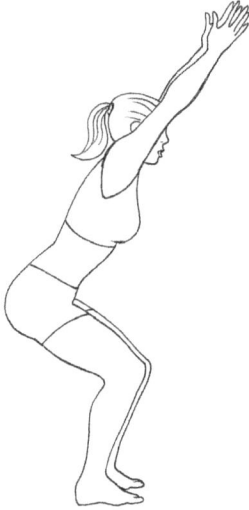

Natalie also calls this the Nile Goddess posture.

As you assume this posture, draw in good energies of your choosing, and release that which no longer works. Be prepared to let the yucky stuff go to make room for the yummy stuff!

In honour of Isis, recite, "The Nile is rising, the Nile is falling, I bring in, and I let go," while maintaining the pose.

Seated Baby Cradle / Mother Mary

Imagine you are holding yourself as a small child in your own arms. Rock this baby that is you. Feel the love emanating from your heart centre as you breathe.

Chant a sweet lullaby as you hold your pose.

"I am loved, I am cradled, I am adored."

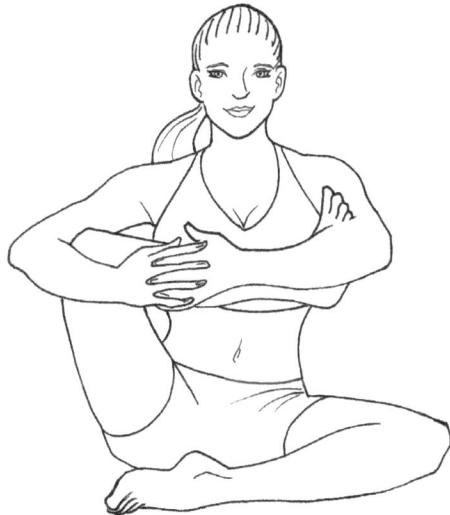

Butterfly / Baddha Konasana / Goddess Dana

In stimulating the abdominal organs and the lower body, this pose helps shift anything you're fed up about.

Release pent-up, harsh or unsaid words and blocked feelings with the chant, "Flow, flow, flow."

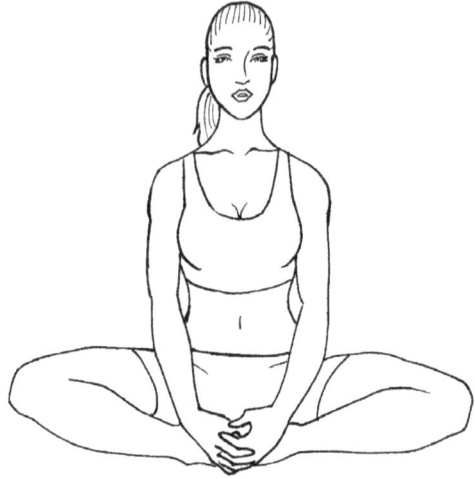

Warrior III / Goddess Isis

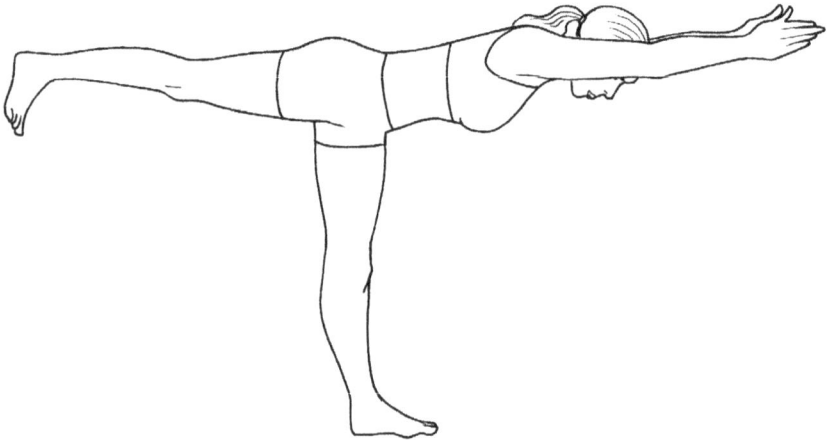

Imagine you are flying high above pain, loss, betrayal and sadness – as well as any pre-wedding blues or jitters! See and trust that everything you're going through is part of life and you will survive!

Chant, "I see, I see, the gift life is meant to be."

Baby Dancer / Nuit Sky Goddess

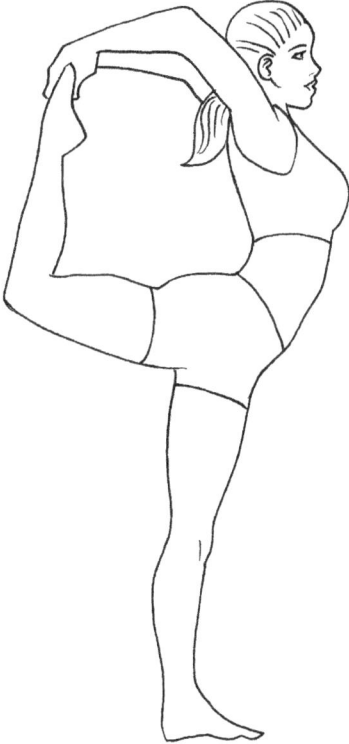

This pose fosters concentration and balance. If you experience difficulty achieving it, listen to your body for answers: what needs to shift in order for new inspiration to enter? Your body already knows the answer – all that is needed is for you to still your mind, and simply, listen, honour and allow.

A suggested affirmation to repeat while maintaining this pose is, "I am eternal, I am free, I'm filled with bliss and harmony!"

If you have trouble holding your pose *and* finding your balance *and* repeating an affirmation, hold onto a chair or the wall for stability.

Again, if you're unfamiliar with yoga, *please seek professional assistance* to help you through each of these poses. A good teacher will also be able to suggest other poses to help you achieve calm. The other advantage of hiring a teacher (several times during your bootcamp!) is that you'll be forced to turn up to your lesson – you won't be able to let yourself get side-tracked by the gadzillion pre-wedding details that steal your valuable "Me Time."

Easy Meditation

Meditation allows you to travel beyond your normal everyday thoughts or thinking patterns and sink deep within a state of relaxation and awareness. Take ten minutes or so to meditate every time you need peace of mind; somewhere quiet that you can escape to inside your head, to reset your thoughts and noise around you. You will be able to calm your mind and find a sense of balance.

Types of Meditation

Breathing Meditation

Breathing meditation will help you relax, calm your breathing, lower your heart rate, and slow your mind from going over and over your wedding checklist.

Find a warm, low-lit, quiet place. Turn on some quiet music. Sit on the floor or in a chair, and get into a comfortable position. I don't recommend you laying down or you may fall asleep, (which, though lovely, is not the goal!) Keep your back straight and start breathing in and out.

Close your eyes partially or completely, and think about cleaning every thought out of your mind. All of the busy – get rid of it – clear everything out. If necessary keep a pen next to you to *write* it out of you, but return to this exercise as soon as you've let the urgent task go. Breathe naturally through your nose. In, out, in out. Just breath normally, but acknowledge your breaths. Think about the actual feeling and sensation of the air going through you. The feeling of the air flowing through your nose and body in general is what your focus will remain on. Don't concentrate on anything else.

Monkey Mind Meditation

If you find that this makes your more fidgety and that your mind is more busy instead of less, don't worry… you are not doing mediation "wrong". You simply have what's known in meditation circles as a monkey mind. One way around this is to simply acknowledge how busy your mind is, without judgement or self-criticism.

Try doing this for ten to fifteen minutes. You will find that your thoughts are subsiding. By the end of your session, you should find yourself more relaxed and energised. Your body has achieved a great sense of calm, and you won't be able to return to a busy mind again immediately.

Wide-Awake Meditation

What if I were to tell you that instead of packing up my yoga mat and warm woolly socks and tottling off to a weekly meditation session, I head to my local café where I do my meditation over coffee? I discovered this form of meditation a few years ago and was so delighted with the results I wrote a book about it![4]

It is an easy meditation style that doesn't require quiet space, or even a quiet mind. In fact, you have permission to have a busy head which helps alleviate any habits of self-criticism for not being able to meditate "right".

---

[4] Wide-Awake Meditation (Now Age Publishing)

Instead of sending your attention inward (as with traditional meditation), Wide-Awake Meditation lets you send your focus outward. It allows you to become highly aware of everything happening around you, become appreciative of the people you meet every day, and to recognise your countless blessings.

If the world inside your head is noisy, cluttered or self-deprecating then you'll probably find the world around you is fractured and confusing. By realigning your focus to seeing a beautiful world, a beautiful world is what you'll manifest. So, quite simply…

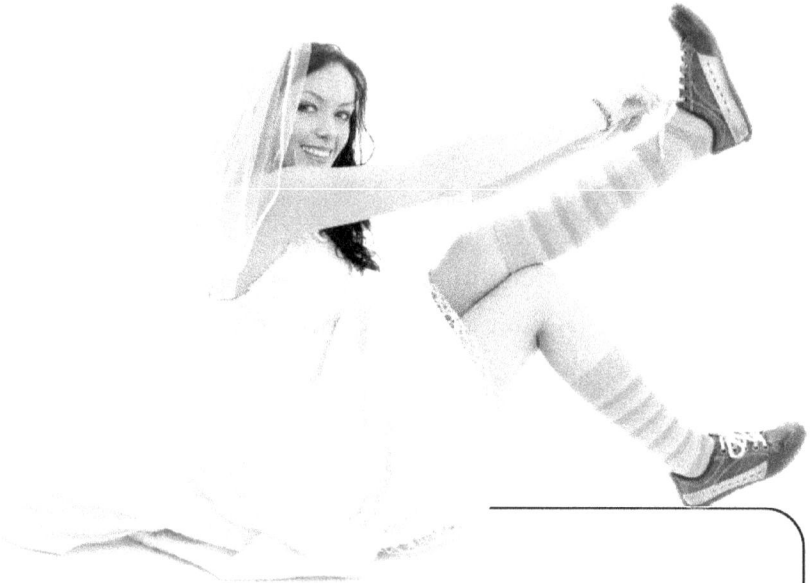

Think beautiful thoughts for a beautiful world.

Delegate! Tasks and Delegation Schedule

Check which tasks you can delegate by ticking them off this list. Write next to each delegated task who you have delegated it to, and when you want them to have it done by.

Of course, you might not need every single bell-and-whistle on this list, in which case, white it out to make it look less intimidating! Remember, **Me Time** is more important than managing every task – stop trying to micro-manage every detail and call on your cheer squad for help.

Apparel

- ☐ Gown _____
- ☐ Bridal shoes _____
- ☐ Bridal lingerie _____
- ☐ Hosiery _____
- ☐ Jewellery _____
- ☐ Headpiece/veil _____
- ☐ Bridesmaid dresses _____
- ☐ Accessories _____
- ☐ Bridesmaid shoes _____
- ☐ Groom's tux _____
- ☐ Groomsmen tuxes _____

- [ ] Garters _____
- [ ] Gown preservation _____
- [ ] Alterations _____
- [ ] Going-away outfit _____
- [ ] Honeymoon clothes _____
- [ ] Flower girl's dress_____
- [ ] Page boy's suit_____

Flowers

- [ ] Brides bouquet _____
- [ ] Bridesmaids bouquets _____
- [ ] Corsages _____
- [ ] Boutonnière _____
- [ ] Reception centerpieces _____
- [ ] Altarpiece _____
- [ ] Pew/chair bows _____
- [ ] Flower girls' flowers _____

Stationary

- [ ] Invitations _____
- [ ] Announcements _____
- [ ] Map/direction cards _____
- [ ] RSVP cards _____
- [ ] Ceremony cards _____
- [ ] Save the date cards _____
- [ ] Postage _____
- [ ] Calligrapher _____

- [ ] Newspaper announce _____
- [ ] Thank you notes _____
- [ ] Rehearsal dinner invites _____
- [ ] Hens invitations _____
- [ ] Hens RSVP and event _____
- [ ] Bachelor party invitations _____
- [ ] Bachelor RSVP and event _____
- [ ] Wedding programs _____
- [ ] Address labels_____
- [ ] Table diagram_____

Ceremony

- [ ] Officiant / Celebrant _____
- [ ] Location hire, permission_____
- [ ] Marriage license (NOIM[5])_____
- [ ] Wedding rings_____
- [ ] Altar decorations _____
- [ ] Chair/pew rental _____
- [ ] Pew/chair decorations _____
- [ ] Certificate signing pen_____
- [ ] Ring bearer pillow _____
- [ ] Flower girl basket _____
- [ ] Unity candle / sand vase_____
- [ ] Ushers_____

---

5 A "Notice Of Intent to Marry" is required in Australia. For step-by-step instructions for getting married in Australia, visit www.GetMarriedInAustralia.com

☐   Transport to service_____

☐   Transport from service_____

☐   Childcare_____

☐   Rice, petals, bubbles_____

Reception and Miscellaneous

☐   Location fee_____

☐   Caterer_____

☐   Food_____

☐   Musician_____

☐   Emcee_____

☐   Bar tender_____

☐   Liquor, mixers, H2O_____

☐   Security_____

☐   Guest book/pen_____

☐   Parking_____

☐   Wedding cake _____

☐   Cake knife, servers_____

☐   Table decorations _____

☐   Other decorations _____

☐   Dishes, Glassware _____

☐   Napkins, Linens_____

☐   Tables, Chairs_____

☐   Parking_____

☐   Wedding favours_____

☐   Hair and make-up_____

Rev Up The Attitude

The Essential Ingredient For Guaranteed Weight Loss

I'm being totally blunt here, but sometimes we've gotta 'lock and load' to get the point across. So, here's the point, point blank: *Holistic well-being is only achievable when you merge the three crucial aspects of body, mind and spirit.* That is, to be successful in unleashing your inner wow-factor, you must look after your body, align your attitude to self-appreciation, and draw on your authentic power within.

As such, this chapter examines *why* it is so important to like yourself in order to achieve the beautiful bride tag you're looking for. A healthy attitude is a vital ingredient in this matrix; it contributes to well-being in so many ways, at so many levels, but let's begin with this little analogy, borrowed from my book, *The Goddess DIET, See a Goddess in the Mirror in 21 Days*.

The woman who stands in front of her mirror every morning and trash-talks her reflection, is the woman who goes to work and pigs out on the morning tea doughnuts.

"I'm fat and ugly anyway," she reminds herself, "six doughnuts won't matter."

Oh, there might be a day when she denies herself any treats as a means of control. But deep down she knows that the more she resists the more she becomes obsessed with the sacrifice and the more likely she will gorge on it later. This woman's attitude is one of self-loathing, and keeps her in the "fat loop".

The woman who stands in front of the mirror and says nice things to her reflection, on the other hand, is pouring self-respect through every cell of her body. This self-respect filters through to her actions and choices through-out the day.

When the doughnuts are put in front of her, she takes only one. She enjoys her first bite because it is a treat, not trash. She may not finish the doughnut, knowing that sometimes, one taste is enough.

This woman's attitude is one of self-appreciation. This is the essential ingredient to easy and permanent weight-loss.

And so, this chapter focuses on your inner beauty and your attitude. Good luck as you embark on this part of your bootcamp – enjoy the tools which will become part of you for life.

Other Tools for Connecting With Your Thinner Goddess

1. Affirmations

An affirmation is a short, positive statement that describes an ideal outcome of a wish or desire. By identifying what you want from your life and expressing it in words as though it has already come to fruition, you are sending a clear message to the Universe of what you want it to provide.

The affirmation you choose must be a dedicated belief, not just an ad hoc approach to "trying it out". Choose an affirmation and work with it dozens of times daily in the lead-up to your wedding. Eventually you will find that because you've committed yourself to making this wish come true, your affirmation will come true.

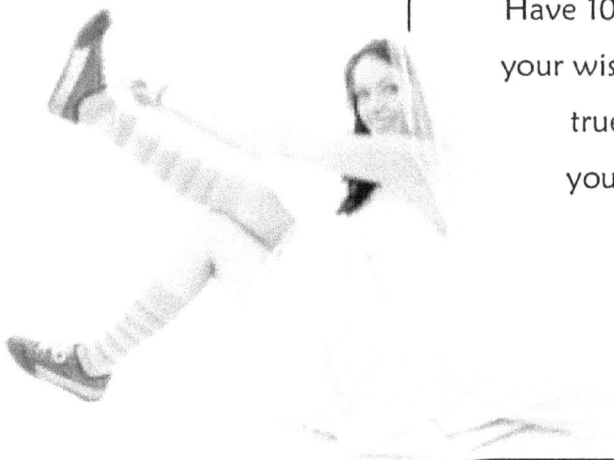

Have 100% faith that your wishes will come true. Believe that you truly deserve what you are asking for.

There are many variations and outcomes possible. They can be spoken out aloud, recorded in your private diary repetitively, written on your computer screen saver, or written on individual sticky notes and hung around your daily environment.

Alternatively, download the bonus poster, choose your favourite affirmation, cut it out and keep it in your wallet. The poster can be downloaded from this secret link:

NowAgePublishing.com/ poster_bootcamp.pdf

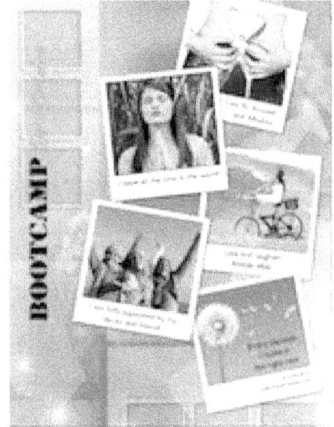

Keys to a Great Affirmation

Imagine that your fairy godmother has granted you a wish. Perhaps you asked to lose weight. Focus on how you feel after the magic wand has been waved and the wish fulfilled. Are you now comfortable in your body and clothes? Are you feeling fitter? Stronger? More alive? Knock-em-dead in that dress? If so, your affirmation could be, "I am a happy, healthy and stunning bride."

Your affirmation should always be written in present tense. Using words like"will do" keeps your outcome in the future out of your reach. It should also be written using positive words – the Universe does not acknowledge negative words such as "not." For example, if you say "I am not poor" the Universe hears "I am poor." Ask instead for, "I have enough money for all that I need."

2. Mirror Work: Getting Real About Loving Your Body

It is a hot topic that the media, fashion houses and society at large perpetuate the myth that a beautiful woman is thin, young and rich. Dove commissioned a study in 2005 and found that out of 3300 girls and women between the ages of 15 and 64 in 10 countries, 68 percent agreed that media and advertising set an unrealistic standard of beauty that they could not hope to achieve. It's important to remember that yes, models are beautiful, but again, they are only one kind of beautiful.

Thankfully the air-brush was unheard of when Rubens, Botticelli and Bouguereau were creating their fabulous works. They have inspired countless modern day works such as Venice Reconstituted at Venice Beach (by California artist Rip Cronk, 1989, pictured next page), or Baron Von Lind's stunning pin-ups, or the alluring burlesque performers that captivate audiences world-wide.

The rubenesque curves and ethereal goddess magnetism is a standard of beauty that you are absolutely capable of achieving. In fact, if you look hard enough in the mirror, I'm sure you'll find elements of the divine in there. In fact, it is a daily requirement of the 7-Day Bootcamp for Brides that you do a few minutes of "Mirror Work" every morning.

Here are some different activities you can do to ditch the old habit of self-criticism and start seeing how beautiful you really are.

Beauty Is As Beauty Does

Begin by looking into a mirror first thing every morning. Hold your own gaze for a short period of time, and say meaningfully, "You are beautiful," or, "Hello goddess." Do not let any negative voice counter-act this statement. If you do hear the inner critic pipe up, repeat the exercise from the start until you feel a little flutter of happiness when you say / hear the words.

Acknowledge Your Beautiful Bits

Where your attention goes, energy flows. Focussing on a spare tyre only adds weight to the issue, (boom boom).

Express gratitude to your beautiful bits by affirming your reflection, and watch these 'bits' take precedence. Suddenly your round tummy is beautiful because you're looking at it with kind eyes.

When you lose attachment to 'ugliness', it loses it grip on you. Your body can then settle into its own perfect size, naturally and beautifully.

Image right: "Venice Reconstituted" Rip Cronk, 1989, at Venice Beach, California. (Photo by Anita Revel)

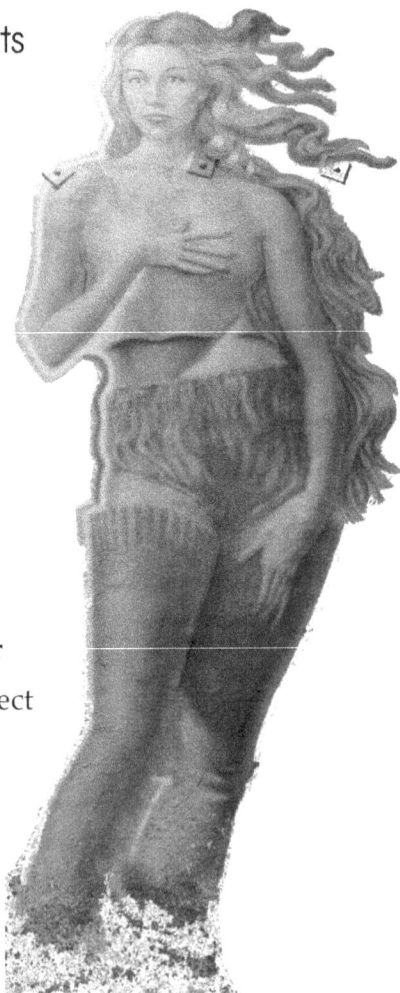

3. Personal Theme Songs

Songs and music have long-been essential tools to help get athletes into a "winner" mindset. Athletes use music to block out internal noise; to help distract them from self-doubt and negative thoughts and instead reprogram their thoughts with positive, upbeat stuff. They often get into a "zone" before they compete using music to help them visualise what they are going to do during their performance.

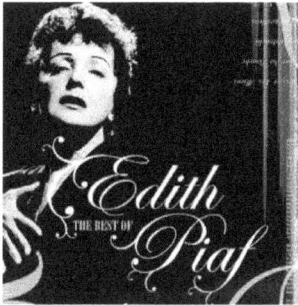

Non, Je Ne Regrette Rien

Edith Piaf

American figure skater, Johnny Weir, listens to Edith Piaf's *Non, Je Ne Regrette Rien* (Regrets I Have None) before competing – there is something poetically beautiful about sweeping away the past, the pains and the pleasures, and "… starting on new bases … because my life, my happiness, today everything begins with you."

How appropriate for you as a bride, too, to have a theme song everyday of your workout to get you into a happy and positive mindset about your pending nuptials.

You could choose a song that is your entry music and visualise how it's going to be walking down that aisle, with friends and family smiling at you, their eyes welling with tears of happiness… already, do you feel happier just thinking about it?

Or you could choose a song that simply makes you feel good. Use it as a crutch for every time you're feeling stressed or overwhelmed slip back into a good space by singing your theme song.

I'm including a list of suggested theme songs to get you started. Some will appeal to your "inner goddess" – that beautiful, sassy, soulful person you were born to be. Others are designed to get you dancing, helping you expel nervous energy. Yet others are simply there just to make you feel good!

At the start of your 7-Day Bootcamp, prepare a list of seven songs (or more!) you think will help you rock your last week as a single woman. Create a playlist and make your iPod and headphones your best friend this week.

Theme Songs for Brides-To-Be

This is a selection of songs that feature in a "Listmania" I created at Amazon.com . I add to the list as brides suggest their favourite theme songs (and are happy to share them). You are welcome to check the Listmania list for updates.

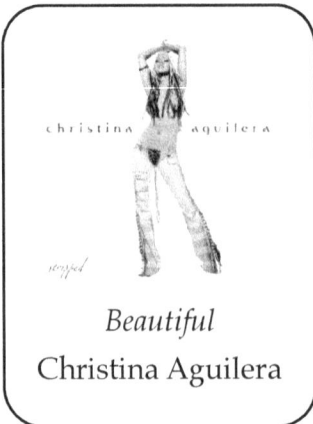

Beautiful
Christina Aguilera

"Cause you are beautiful; beautiful in every single way," sings Christina Aguilera. Every bride needs a personal uplifter for times when she is doubting herself, or having fears her dress won't fit, or perhaps because of a pre-marital tiff that has got her down. Christina reminds you that – girl, you are beautiful!

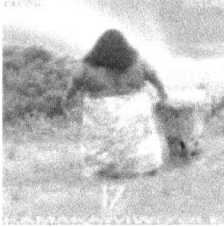

Over the Rainbow
Iz Kamakawiwo'ole

Israel Kamakawiwo'ole's version of *Over the Rainbow* features in movie soundtracks such as *Finding Forrester*, *Meet Joe Black* and *50 First Dates* for a reason – it is bright, uplifting and just makes a girl feel super happy! You'll be dreaming of Hawaii, blue skies and *love* before the song is even half-way through.

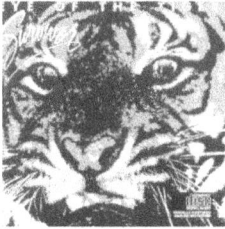

Eye of the Tiger
Survivor

I haven't met a bride yet who doesn't want to look toned in her wedding dress. This is the song that rocked Rocky Balboa through his punishing-yet-rewarding training regimes. Likewise it will help you push through yet another set of sit-ups, push-ups and epic stair-climbs. You can do it sister!

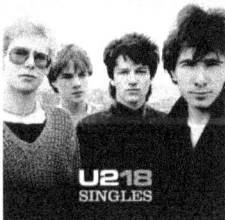

Beautiful Day
U2

For days when you wake up and the clouds are grey, the stress is building, the doubts are creeping in… This song by Irish super group U2, will help turn your focus from doom-and-gloom to a positive outlook. Suddenly, by focusing on a beautiful day, your day actually becomes one.

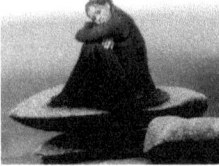

You Gotta Be
Des'ree

Got an interfering mother-in-law? Or a pushy wedding planner over-riding your decisions? Here's your theme song to give you courage… "… You gotta be cool, you gotta be calm, You gotta stay together…" and once you've regained your centre, well, "All I know, all I know, love will save the day."

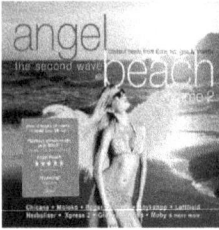

Breathe
Mulsanne

Every bride needs time out from the chaos surrounding her in the lead-up to the wedding. *Breathe* is the perfect track from the *Angel Beach* album to help you take five minutes and simply… *breathe*… Actually, the whole album is worth a listen, especially when five minutes of bliss just isn't enough.

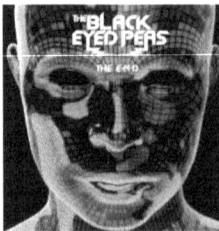

I Gotta Feeling
Black-Eyed Peas

The months of planning, the weeks of panic, the days of a thousand last details – the Big Day is here. Do you want your mood to be… "Has the salmon arrived, do the napkins match the plates, is Grandpa Grumpypants behaving…?" or do you want it to be "Tonight's gonna be a good, GOOD NIGHT!"?

The Bootcamp for Life: Fabulosity Forever

The 7-Day Bootcamp For Brides is a seven-day program for jumping-into-high-gear, shedding-some-last-minute-inches, toning-some-muscles-for-the-dress and taking-some-much-needed-Me-Time.

It's designed to help you cope with an intense time of your life in the safest way and in the shortest way possible. Follow it and you will protect yourself from the typical stress-ridden, starvation-rife, sleepless week that many brides go through.

However, did you know…

… You can apply the principles of the bootcamp for a **lifetime of health and happiness**? To remind you, it's all about the Four Rs…

1. **Real Food** – Eat natural, unprocessed foods, and follow the Real Food Rules:
    1. Eat slowly,
    2. Complement your foods,
    3. Eat early, and
    4. Detox and cleanse

2. **Recreation**;
3. **Re-Hydration**, and
4. **Rest**

Get your Four Rs priority in your life and bang, you have guaranteed:

- ✓ Weight regulation,
- ✓ Regular energy burn,
- ✓ Even moods,
- ✓ Focus and clarity,
- ✓ Day in, day out, *fabulosity*!

So resolve to stick with the Four Rs for life and you'll be golden! Continue using the Companion worksheets included in this book until your new habits are well-and-truly ingrained. You'll know you've succeeded when it's easier to *do* the new habit rather than *not* do it.

Good luck, and I hope your wedding day is every bit as wonderful as you intend it to be. Shine on!

Appendix

Resources: Books, Articles, Social Media & Other Services

Resources

✓ The Australian government recommend 2.5 hours of moderate exercise a week. Download the guidelines: ausport.gov.au/fulltext/1999/feddep/physguide.pdf

✓ The United States Department of Agriculture has a comprehensive online database of nutrient profiles for 13,000 foods. You can find them under "Food and Nutrition" at usda.gov

Recommended Books

✓ *The Goddess DIET, See a Goddess in the Mirror in 21 Days*
~ Anita Revel (Now Age Publishing)

✓ *Goddess Makeover, a Home-Study Course in Personal Values, Self-Actualisation and Divine Revellion*
~ Anita Revel (Now Age Publishing)

eBooks

✓ *DIY Wedding Bible*
~ Maggie Magee (Now Age Publishing)

✓ *BOTIBOTO, Beautiful On The Inside Beautiful On The Outside, An Empowerment Story for Well-Rounded Women*
~ Anita Revel (Now Age Publishing)

Articles

✓ How to Write Your Wedding Vows. Read the article at ehow.com/how_5937438_write-wedding-vows.html

✓ Step-by-step guide: How to Get Married in Australia: GetMarriedInAustralia.com

Social Media

✓ Anita Revel's Civil Marriage Celebrancy on Twitter: @YesIDoWeddings

✓ Anita Revel on Facebook: facebook.com/AnitaRevel

✓ The Goddess Diet on Facebook: facebook.com/TheGoddessDiet

Services

✓ Anita Revel: Civil Marriage Celebrant / Officiant in Australia and America: YesIDoWeddings.com

✓ Melanie Grace: Personal Fitness Coach / Miracle Endorphins: MiracleEndorphins.com

✓ Natalie Maisel: Californian yoga teacher, moon mistress and workshop leader: GoddessDowload.com

About the Author

As described on Anita's website (AnitaRevel.com), Anita is a creatrix, author, mother and wife, web diva, dream weaver, lover of life. She's also a Civil Marriage Celebrant, teacher, artist, traveller and joy junkie but couldn't make these rhyme.

Nevertheless, all these roles sum up her passion for inspired living. As such, her work helps you connect with your beautiful, sassy, intuitive, lovable, sacred and authentic Self – your inner goddess.

Anita is also the author of a growing collection of well-being resources in various forms of manifestation, countless columns for United Press International, hundreds of articles found sprinkled across the internet, and numerous books for women's well-being.

Anita lives on a farm in the stunning Margaret River region of Western Australia with her husband, two children and a dog as loyal as his nearest cuddle.

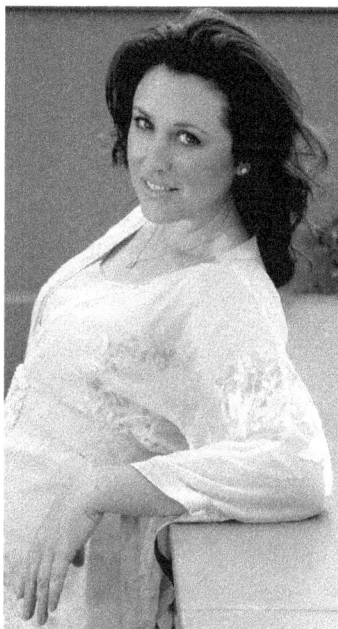